# 269 RED HOT XXX *Rated* QUESTIONS

## *Super Sexy Ticklers to Tempt, Tease and Spark*

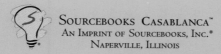

SOURCEBOOKS CASABLANCA™
AN IMPRINT OF SOURCEBOOKS, INC.®
NAPERVILLE, ILLINOIS

Published by Sourcebooks Casablanca, an imprint of Sourcebooks, Inc.
P.O. Box 4410, Naperville, Illinois 60567-4410
(630) 961-3900
Fax: (630) 961-2168
www.sourcebooks.com

ISBN-13: 978-1-4022-0894-2
ISBN-10: 1-4022-0894-4

Printed and bound in the United States
DR 10 9 8 7 6 5 4 3 2 1

# INTRODUCTION

Can you ever know enough about what turns your lover on? What makes them a seething hot bundle of passion, and what turns them cold as a sleety day in January? Here are 269 questions you can use to unlock each other's secret fantasies, share favorites that are closest to your hearts, and explore tantalizing new ways to play. What better way to get hot and heavy with your lover than to cuddle up and answer these steamy questions? Use them to build anticipation, come up with new ideas for red-hot sex, or just have a sexy good time.

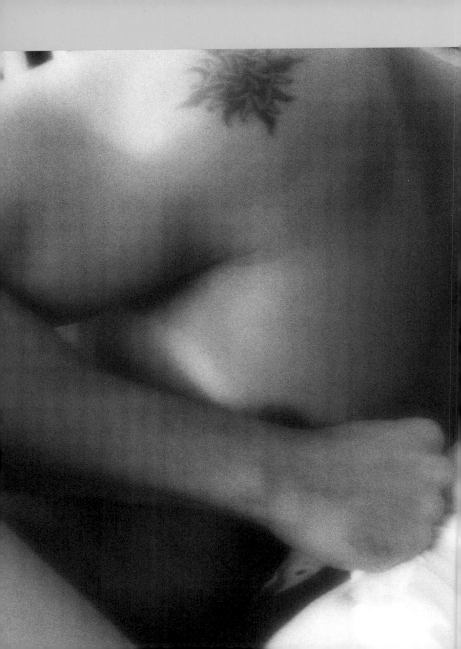

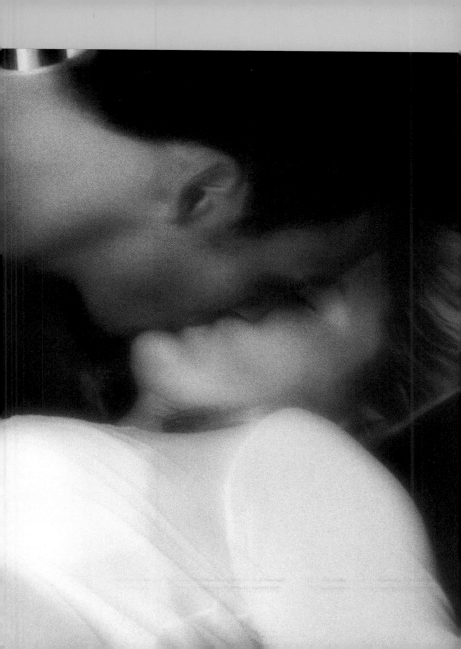

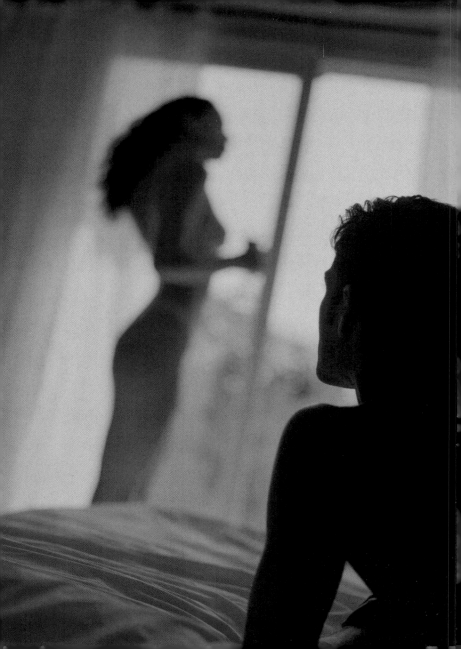

# FORBIDDEN FANTASIES

I know you have untapped depths of passion. Tell me, in detail, any sexual fantasy you've always wanted to try—maybe that forbidden thing isn't out of the question.

1  Is there any desire that you want to try that you think is taboo?

2  Is there an outfit you'd love to wear but haven't because you're afraid I'd think it was too weird?

3  Are there any new positions you wanted to try but are too shy to ask me? I'm game!

4 Do you have any sexual fetishes that you want to explore?

5 Do you think sexual fantasies should stay fantasies or be made reality?

6 Are there any secret desires you've never told anyone?

7 Will you tell me?

# EITHER/OR

Having to choose between one scenario or the other is exciting and satisfying—and you can always go back another time and test the other option!

8    If you could spy on me through the crack of the door, which would you rather witness—me touching myself, or taking a long, steamy shower?

9    Which would you rather have for your afternoon delight—a lunchtime quickie, or a quick conversation so hot it melts the phone lines?

**10** If it was too hot to wear clothes, would we play strip poker, or sit in front of the open refrigerator and play with ice cubes?

**11** Which would you rather have—me stripping very seductively and very slowly while you watched or coming home to find me already naked on the bed waiting for you?

**12** If I woke you up using my mouth, would you keep your eyes closed and let me have my way with you or would you wake up and join me in my efforts?

# I'M SEEING PORN STARS

Let's discuss what our roles would be if we were a part of the growing adult movie industry (and see if we can't make something of our own grow).

**13** What do you think you would be famous for if you were a porn star?

**14** What do you think I would be famous for if I were a porn star?

**15** What porn star name would you invent for me?

**16** What kind of porn movie would we make together (kinky, funny, or classy)?

**17**  When can we make that porn movie?

**18**  What's your favorite XXX-rated movie?

**19**  Would you watch your favorite porn movie with me?

**20**  Would you test out some of the techniques we saw or would you be too shy?

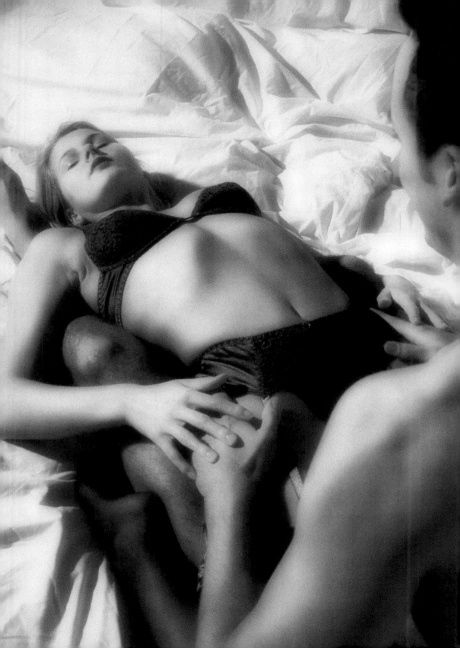

# FAVORITES!

Learn which tantalizing tidbits of your sex life are your lover's favorites and create some new ones.

21 What is your favorite erotic memory of me?

22 What is your favorite sexy part of me?

23 Outside the bedroom, what is your favorite household location to have sex?

24 What is your favorite thing about our lovemaking?

**25**    What is your favorite sexual setting?

**26**    What is your favorite music to make love to?

**27**    What is your favorite position?

**28**    What is your favorite role-playing fantasy?

# WOULD YOU, COULD YOU?

You'll never know if you don't ask!

**29** Would you ever go skinny dipping?

**30** Could we have sex fully clothed?

**31** Would you ever work out in the nude?

**32** Could we have sex on the bench press?

**33** Would you ever sit in the back row of a risqué movie and fool around?

**34** Could we make our own risqué movie?

**35** Would you be interested in conducting one red-hot photo session?

**36** Could we look at sensual sculptures and photography from an art book together in bed?

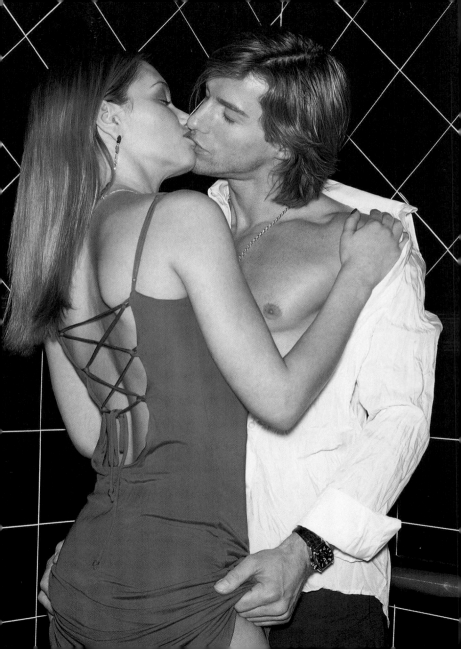

# PUBLIC DISPLAYS OF AFFECTIONS

Let's experience the excitement of being outside and the thrill of getting caught.

37   Oops, I dropped my fork. Would you ever go down on me under the table at a restaurant?

38   Would you be willing to go out without underwear and find a way to do it in public without anyone knowing?

39   Where would you take me to have sex in public?

**40** Would you ever have sex while at work?

**41** Would you have sex in the corner at a department store?

**42** Would you like to make love outside in the rain?

# TEASE ME, READ TO ME

Hearing those riveting words coming from your lips will make me tremble with excitement.

**43** If I bring my favorite erotica to bed, will you bring yours?

**44** I've got an idea for a wildly erotic story—will you help me write it?

**45** Can we put a sexy spin on our favorite classic literature—if I were Juliet, would you plunge your dagger into me?

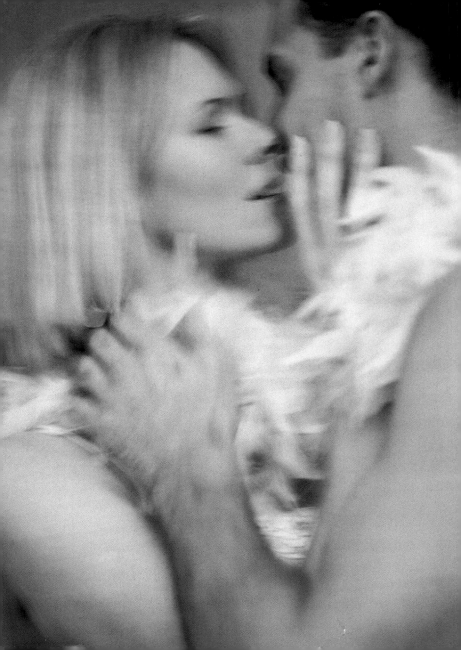

# FANTASY ISLAND

Let's treasure our sex life and reward our-selves with a little booty.

**46** If you were on a deserted island, what one sex prop would you need (besides me)?

**47** If I were to send you on a sexual scavenger hunt throughout the house to find the treasure, would you participate?

**48** I've hidden some honey somewhere on my body. With your tongue, do you think you can find it?

**49** Give me clues to the treasure. Would you create a map of your body and indicate where and when you'd like to be touched during sex?

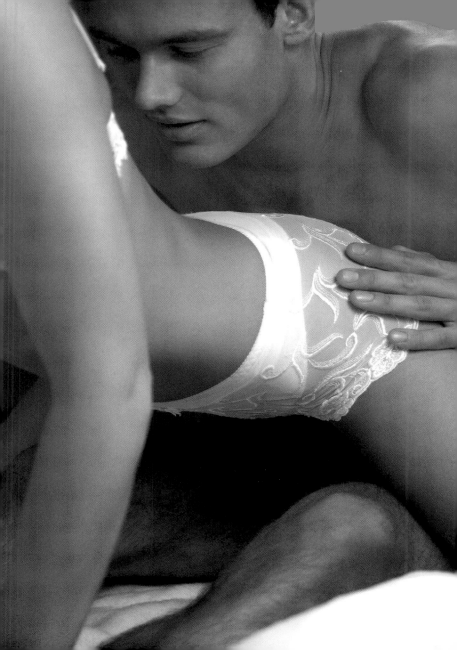

# MOVIE MAGIC

The motion picture industry doesn't have anything on the lusty level of our picture-perfect desire, but it can inspire us to make some magic of our own.

**50** If you were to fantasize that I was a celebrity, who would I be?

**51** If you were to fantasize that you were a celebrity, who would you be?

**52** What movie makes you incredibly horny?

**53** What is your favorite erotic scene from any movie?

## 54 Can we act out your favorite passionate movie scene?

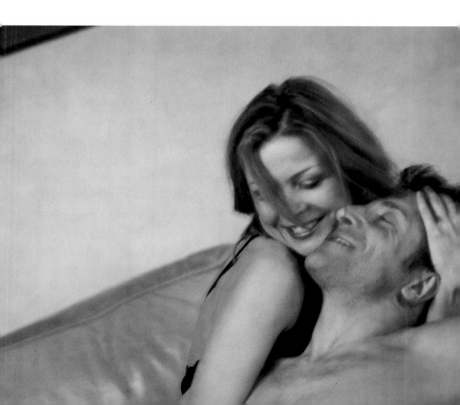

# STEAMY SCENARIOS FOR HER

Make his cheeks blush and his head spin with these heated questions.

55   Gee, I'm feeling a little hoarse—do you have something I can suck on?

56   Would you let me knead gently on your back in my stiletto heels?

57   Would you let me bring a vibrator into our love making as an added stimulant?

58   How would you like me to pay homage to your penis?

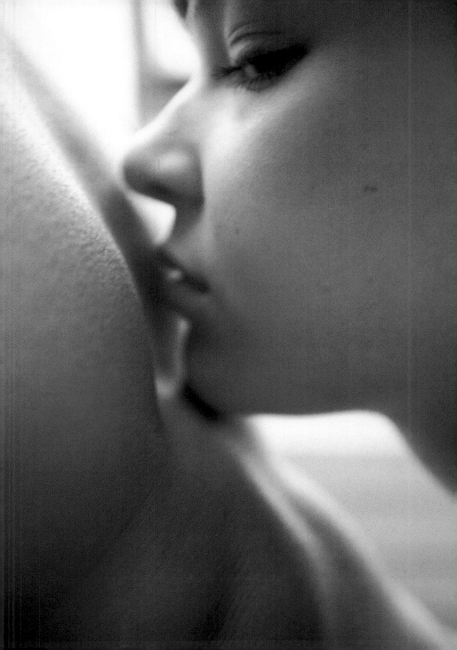

# STEAMY SCENARIOS FOR HIM

Women want to make sure you're always listening. Ask her these questions, and be sure to pay very close attention to the answers.

**59** If we went dancing and I got an erection, would you finish me off in a quiet corner?

**60** What is the highest number of orgasms you've had in one sex romp?

**61** How many do you wish I could give you?

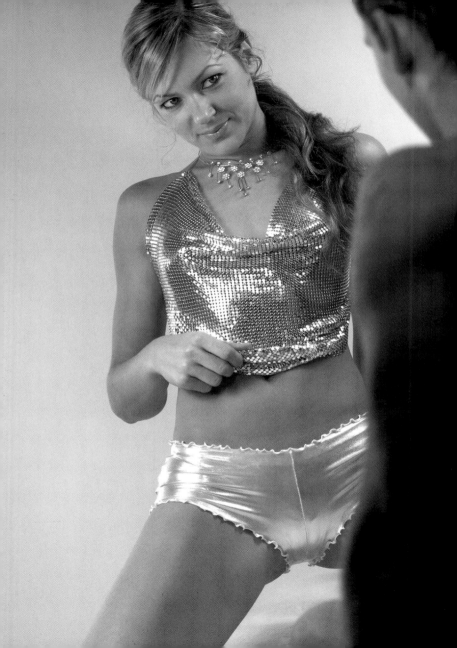

# PLAYING GAMES

It's true that men and women communicate on different wavelengths, but answer these questions and you two will be on the same bed sheet in no time.

**62** Would you ever switch gender roles with me during sex?

**63** Would you ever switch our clothing as well?

**64** What shape do you most enjoy trimmed down there?

**65** If I pick something sexy for you to wear out for the evening, will you pick out something for me?

**66** If we were to let our primitive natures take over and pretend to be animals mating, what species would we be?

**67** Are there any little tricks you'd like me to know about?

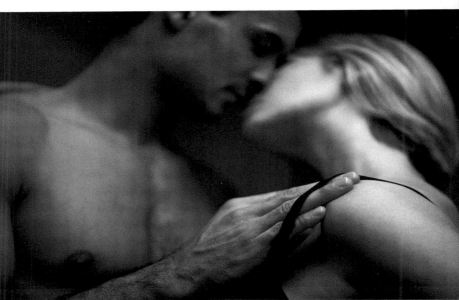

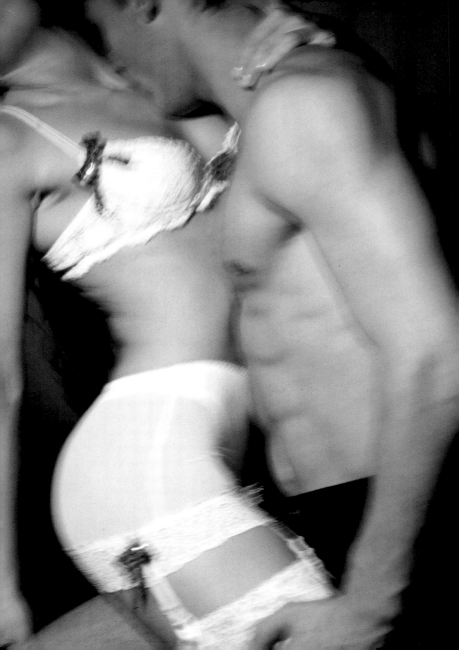

# SHOPPING SEXCAPADES

Get the charge cards ready!—If just asking questions about sex turns us on, imagine how hot and bothered we'll get if we shop in preparation for it.

**68** Can we go on a bed and bath shopping spree? (Egyptian cotton sheets anyone?)

**69** Can't wait to have me until we get home? Would you ever take me in a dressing room to have sex?

**70** Will you go shopping for sexy lingerie with me?

**71** Would you like to just sit in bed, thumbing through a racy lingerie catalog, and pick out some outfits for a little visual stimulation?

**72** Can we go to an XXX-rated store?

**73** Would you be nervous or excited in a sex shop? Or a little bit of both?

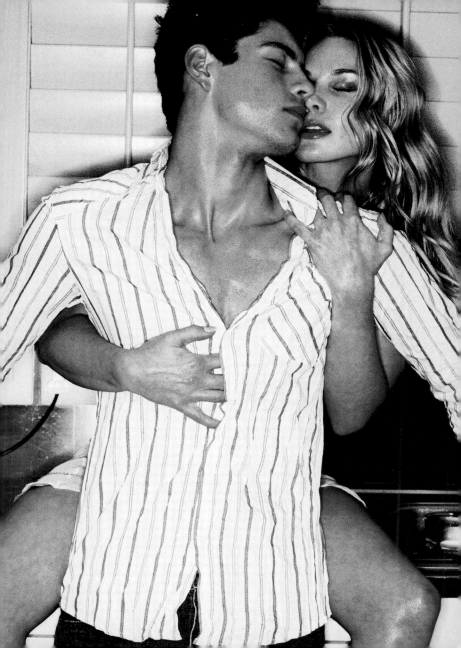

# THE SOUNDS OF SEX

The yelling. The screaming. The moaning. It's all music to our ears. These questions will help you determine if you want it loud and dirty or soft and sweet. Or maybe a musical note in between.

**74** What sounds do you love to hear during sex?

**75** What sounds do you wish I made during sex?

**76** What words do you love to hear during sex?

**77** What would you like me to yell out during my orgasm?

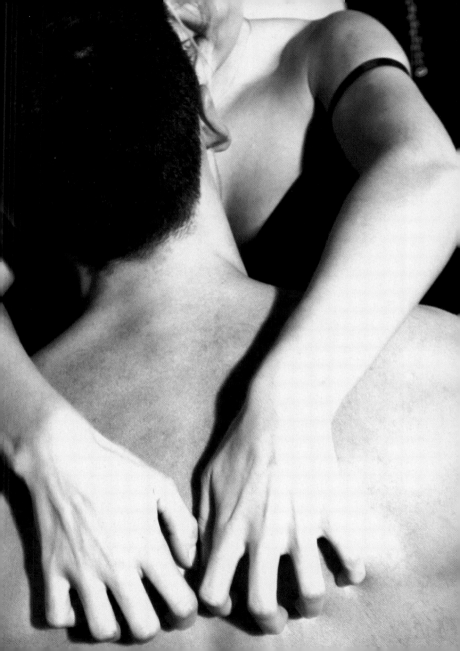

# NUMEROLOGY

Sex should be about *how good* instead of *how much,* but sometimes we're greedy and we want both quality and quantity.

**78** How many times in a week would you like to have sex?

**79** Do you want to try the 69 position?

**80** Wanna find out how many positions we can do in five minutes?

**81** What are your top three favorite positions?

**82** What are the top three erogenous zones on your body?

**83** What do you think are my top three erogenous zones?

**84** How far can we get through the Kama Sutra before we explode?

**85** On a scale of one to ten, how would you rate our lovemaking?

**86** On a scale of one to ten, how would you rate me as a lover?

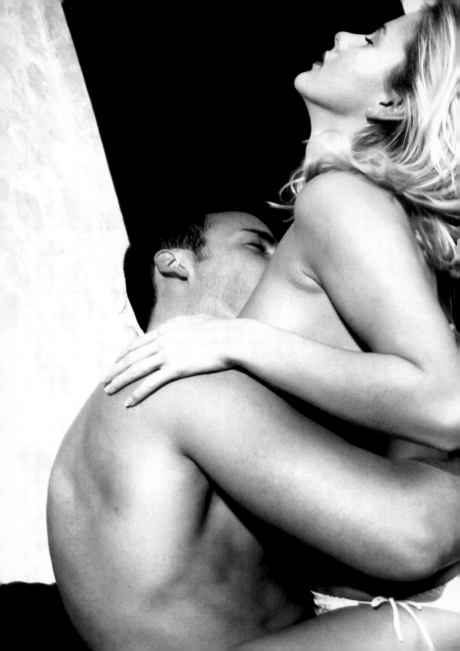

# SHOW AND TELL

How do you want it? Tell me your preferences and I'll tell you mine.

87    Top or bottom?

88    Bedroom or other room?

89    Lights on or off?

90    Public or private?

91    Partially naked or entirely naked?

**92** Oils and lotion or candles and Egyptian cotton sheets?

**93** Naughty videos or hot photographs?

**94** Shaved or *au naturale*?

**95** Lacy panties/silk boxers or leather?

**96** Fast and hard or slow and gentle?

**97** Whipped cream and chocolate or fruit and honey?

**98** Spanking or handcuffs?

**99** Standing up or lying down?

**100** Soft or firm touch?

**101** Under the covers or on top?

**102** Massage from top to bottom or bottom to top?

# LIGHTS! CAMERA! ACTION!

Who do you want to be tonight? Dress me up in whatever costume you desire. Just promise to undress me when the script calls for it.

**103** Pirate and wench?

**104** Seventeenth-century king and his mistress?

**105** French maid and naughty butler?

**106** Master/mistress and slave?

**107** Tarzan and Jane?

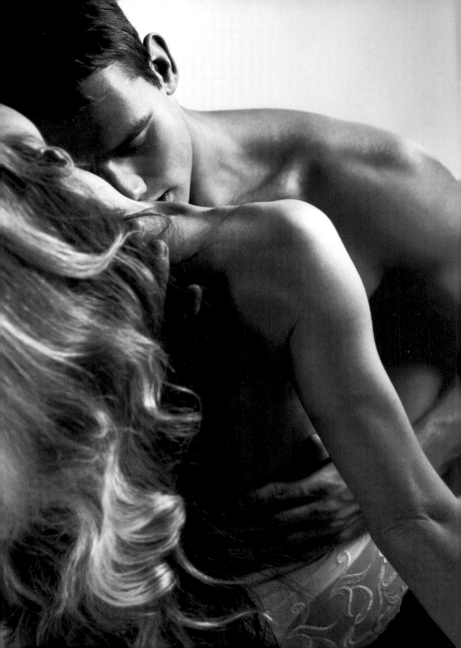

# BE CARNALLY CREATIVE

How far can our imaginations take us? Let's get the creative juices flowing. Other juices are sure to follow.

**113** How would you incorporate scarves into our lovemaking if you could do anything with them—other than tie me up?

**114** How would you give me a back massage without using your hands?

**115** How would you turn me on without touching me at all?

**116** What things can we do with ice cubes besides suck on them?

**117** If you were handcuffed, which body parts would you use to touch me during sex that you would normally use your hands for?

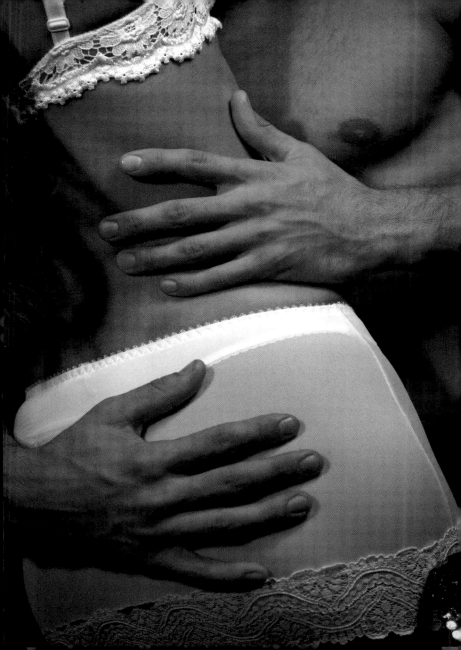

# RANDY REQUESTS

Get what you've always wanted but never had the courage to ask for. Now's the time to live out your deepest carnal fantasies!

**118** Can you please keep the stilettos/boots on?

**119** How about keeping a skirt on with no underwear?

**120** Will you say something really kinky to me while we're making love?

**121** Will you pinch me until it hurts so good?

**122** How about biting me? Or pulling my hair?

**123** Can we incorporate a little light bondage into our sex romp?

**124** Would you book a motel room during our lunch hour?

**125** Would you ever consider a threesome?

**126** Do you want to bring sex toys into the bedroom?

# TEMPT ME! TRUST ME!

You trust your lover with many of your intimate emotions and secrets. Now trust them with all of your luscious body.

**127** Do you trust me enough to close your eyes and let me have my way with you?

**128** Would you let me tie you up with silk scarves?

**129** Do you trust me enough to let me shave you anywhere I want?

**130** Would you trust yourself to keep your concentration if I serviced you while you were driving?

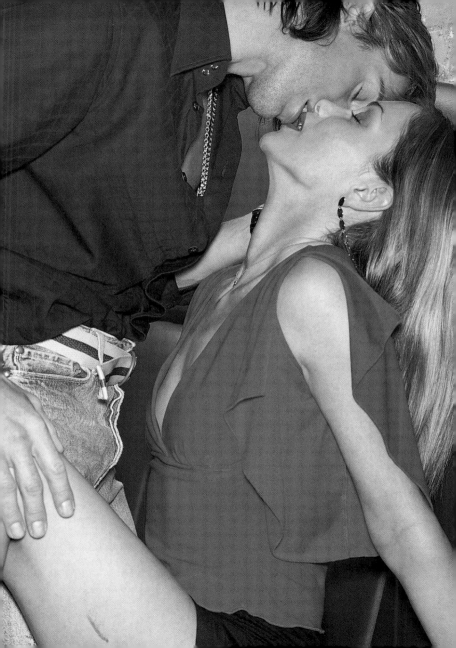

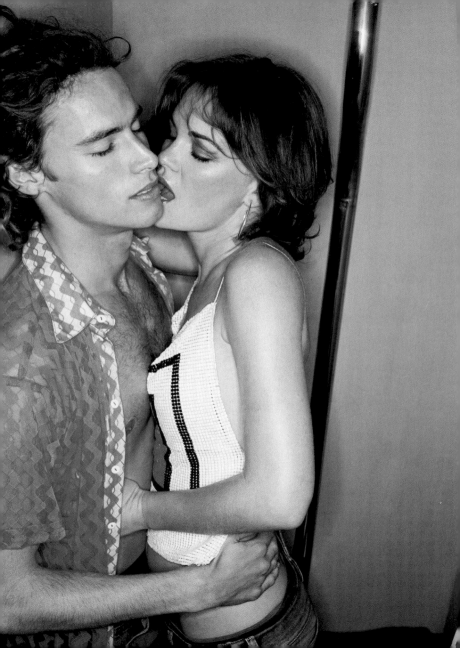

# COMING HOME

Let the innocence of your youth melt away with these hot and steamy questions sure to bring a whole new meaning to the phrase "young at heart."

**131** Would you ever have sex in your childhood bedroom?

**132** Have you ever hooked up on a swing set?

**133** What childhood game would you like to put an adult twist on?

**134** Do you remember one of your first good erotic experiences?

**135** Will you recreate one of your early erotic experiences with me?

**136** Is there something we used to do in our early romping days that you would love to do again?

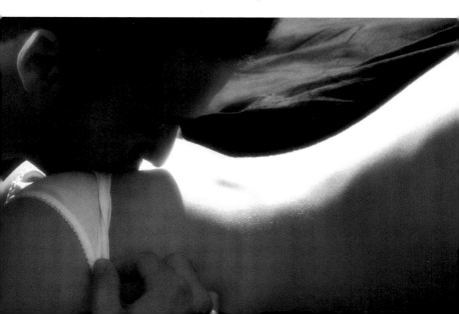

# GETTING TO KNOW YOU

I want you to know all there is to know. Ask me these questions and I'll reveal my innermost secrets as well as my naughty side.

**137** Do you know where my G-spot is?

**138** Do you want me to show you my G-spot?

**139** Will you let me guide your hands so you know exactly what I want?

**140** Will you guide my hands so I know exactly what you want?

**141** Are there any little tricks you'd like me to know?

**142** What is it that you absolutely need sexually?

**143** What is something that you've always wanted?

**144** Do you promise to tell me when you have a new idea for us to try out?

**145** What do you like best about our lovemaking?

**146** What is the most sexually mysterious thing about me?

**147** What is something you've never done in bed before?

**148** Do you ever feel misunderstood by the opposite sex? How can I help?

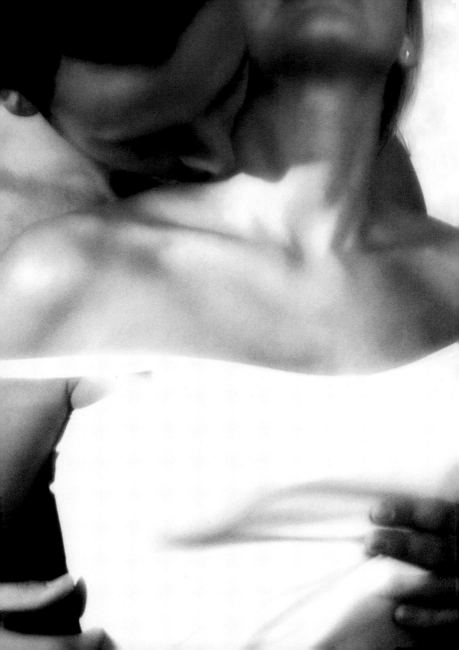

# IT'S ALL IN THE TIMING

It seems we never spend enough time doing the very important things. Let's set aside the calendars and cell phones for a full afternoon and see what comes up.

**149** For you, what is the sexiest time of year?

**150** What time of day would you prefer to have sex?

**151** How long do you think our orgasms last? Can we time them?

**152** How quick can we make our quickie?

**153** How long can we make one lovemaking session last?

**154** If we wear as little as possible without touching, how long do you think we'll last until temptation takes over?

**155** How long can we just kiss until our hands begin to wander?

# ILLICIT INTIMACIES

Let's indulge in the intimate acts that are ours alone—then let's make up a few new ones!

**156** What sexual act do I do that you cannot live without?

**157** What would you name our favorite position?

**158** What do you consider your special talents in bed?

**159** What do you consider my special talents in bed?

**160** What do you absolutely need to see that turns you on?

**161** Do we have a sexual cue for when we are in public and absolutely need to go home?

**162** If not, can we create a signal that's ours alone?

**163** Would you promise to always tell me exactly what you want while we're making love?

**164** What do you think is your signature move?

**165** What is my signature move?

**166** When and where was the best orgasm I ever gave you?

**167** If blindfolded, could you tell the right side of my chest from my left side?

# HORNY HOLIDAYS

The holidays are extra special for everyone—a time set aside to show your love and devotion. A perfect opportunity to show off your randy side.

**168** If I were Cupid, would you let me shoot off my arrow?

**169** If I dressed up as a bunny for Easter, would you cover me in chocolate and nibble at my ears?

**170** On Thanksgiving, in honor of being thankful for reaching uncharted land, will you take a pilgrimage to discover new territory on my body?

**171** On the Fourth of July, can we lie underneath the fireworks and make our own explosions? We'll celebrate with a bang!

**172** If I dressed up as Santa would you sit on my lap and tell me what you want for Christmas?

**173** Would you put your candle in my jack-o'-lantern?

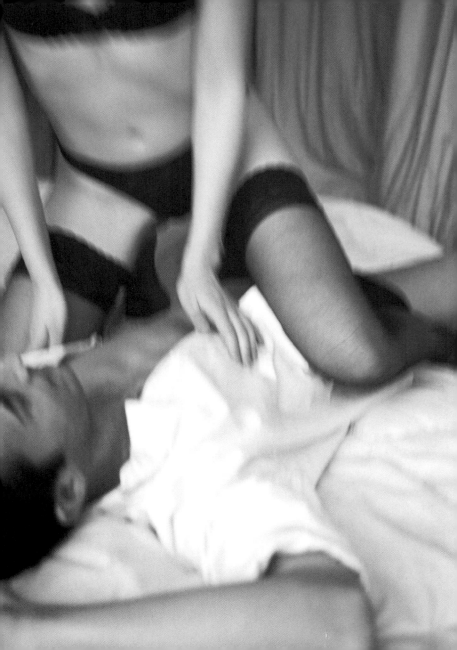

# RANDOM RANDY QUESTIONS

The best questions are the ones that come from nowhere. The best answers are the ones that make you come undone.

**174** I've been bad — how will you punish me?

**175** Do you want me to take control? I'll take care of everything.

**176** How could we spice up our sex life?

**177** Are you willing to take a little risk?

**178** Are you in the mood for a little light bondage?

**179** I have an interesting scenario in my mind—want to play?

**180** What do you want to be tonight?

**181** If you could beg me for anything, what would it be?

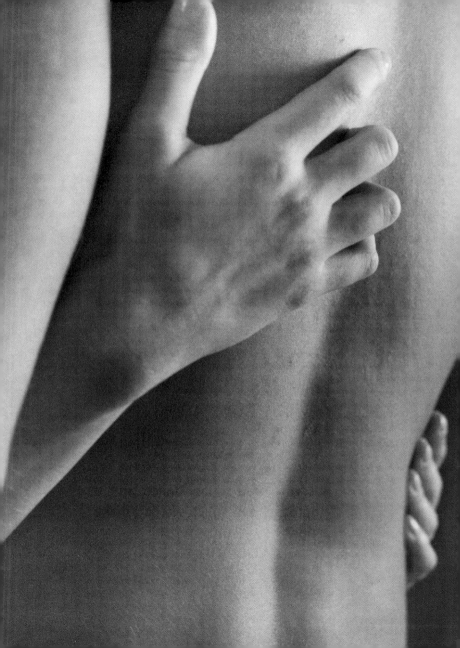

# ENDLESS EROTIC POSSIBILITIES

These tantalizing questions deal with the could-haves, should-haves, and what-ifs of our sex life. Let's see if our answers can make these possibilities a rewarding reality.

**182** If someone was in the next room while we made love, would it make you nervous or excited?

**183** If we had a mirror by the bed, would you watch us as we made love, or watch me?

**184** If I gave you a lap dance and a striptease, how much would I make in tips?

**185** Are you ready to find out just how talented a dancer I am?

**186** Would you ever have sex discreetly at a concert? (How about indiscreetly?)

**187** Have you ever gone to a nude beach? Would you?

**188** Would you join the crowd and take off your bathing suit?

**189** Would it bother you if I got naked at the beach?

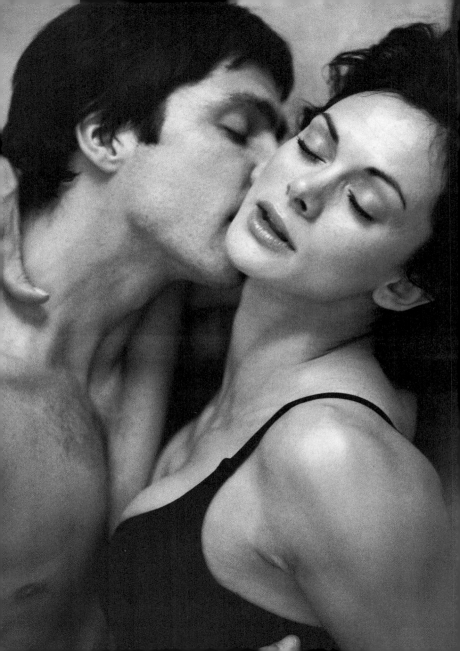

# SENSE AND SENSUALITY

The five senses are an essential part of living life richly. Let's discover how essential they are to a richly delicious sex life.

**190** Do you close your eyes when you have an orgasm, or do you look at me?

**191** What body parts do you watch while we have sex?

**192** What is your favorite place for me to touch while you come?

**193** What is my signature scent?

**194** Can you tell me what my skin tastes like? My lips? My most intimate places?

**195** How would you describe the scent of our lovemaking?

**196** What sounds do I make during sex that turn you on the most?

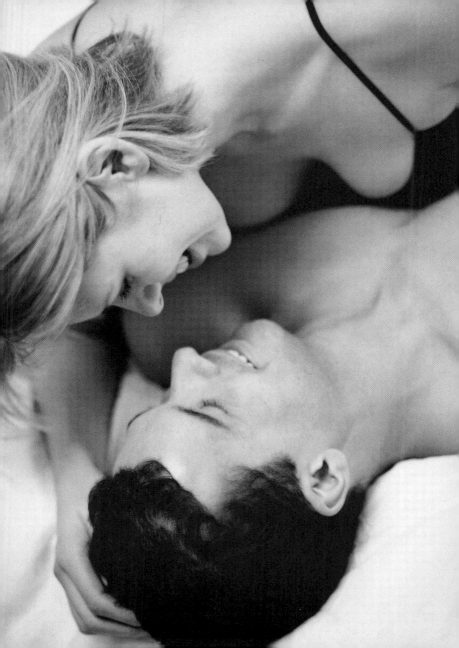

# LET'S EXPERIMENT

Eureka! Let's conduct some experiments. With a little trial and error we'll get all the right kinds of explosions!

**197**  Can you orgasm by nipple stimulation alone?

**198**  Can you orgasm by testicle stimulation alone?

**199**  Are you up for an experimental kissing session? Anything goes, anywhere!

**200**  Can we focus on the sexual act itself without worrying about finishing with an orgasm?

# GETTING DOWN AND DIRTY

Let's travel down that treasure trail on the road to pleasure town.

**201** Are you willing to put marshmallows in your mouth before oral sex?

**202** How about switching from hot tea to ice cubes?

**203** Will you suck on a strong mint while you give me oral sex?

**204** How about a hand job? Blow job? Lube job?

**205** Would you like to tell me your most secret sensitive place? I'll promise to touch you deeply.

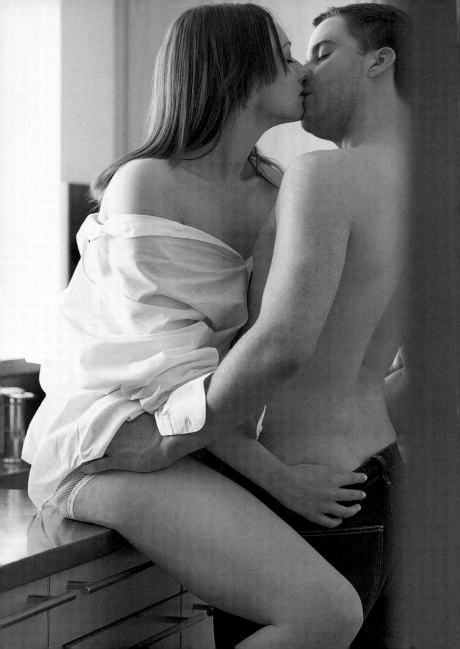

# MOUTH-TO-MOUTH COLLISION

I'll waive your ticket in exchange for some community service—lessons in kissing all the right places.

**206** Where would you like to be kissed that I've never kissed before?

**207** How important to you is kissing?

**208** Where would you kiss me deeply if my mouth was off limits?

**209** Can you describe to me your first kiss?

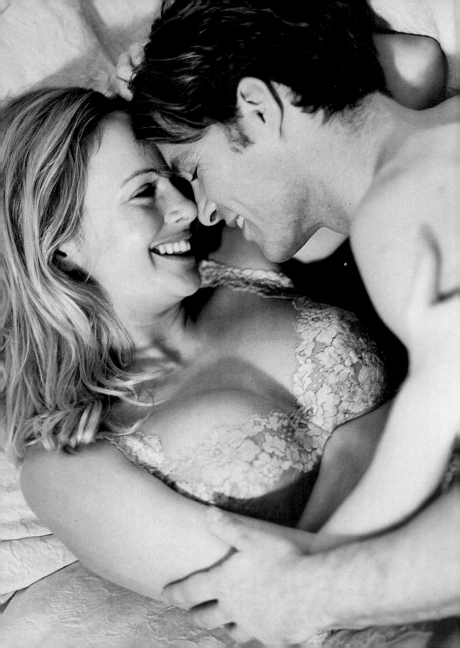

# SEXUALLY SINCERE

Honesty is truly the best sexual policy and allows for our emotions and our bodies to be orgasmically open!

**210** Have you ever faked an orgasm?

**211** Do you take care of yourself when I'm not around?

**212** What are some of the fantasies you imagine while you're doing it?

**213** Can I watch you do it?

**214** What is your most ticklish spot?

**215** Are you self-conscious about any part of your body?

216    Is there any time you've felt vulner-able during sex?

217    Do you have any sexual regrets?

218    If a lover ever cheated on you, would you take them back?

219    How important is sex in your life?

220    How important is love in your life?

221    Can you describe the orgasm I give you?

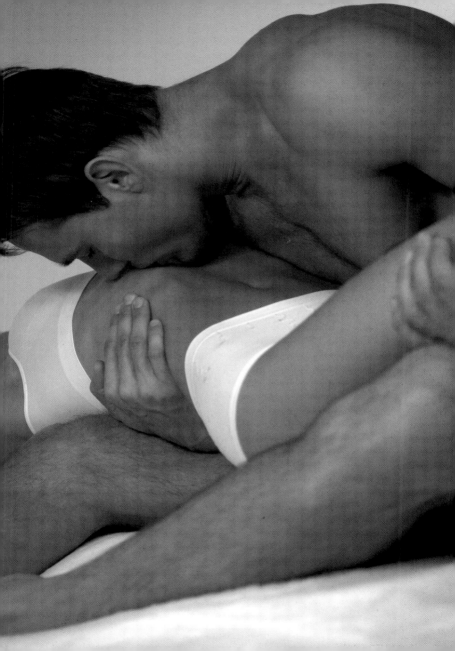

# CARNAL HISTORY

Our sexual background defines who we once were and who we have become. Ask these probing questions and discover who you'll soon be coming into.

222 What was the biggest fight you've ever had with a lover?

223 Do you believe in the healing power of make-up sex?

224 Have you ever told a complete stranger something that you've held back from a lover?

**225**  Have you ever had a one-night stand?

**226**  Have you ever rebounded and known you were doing so?

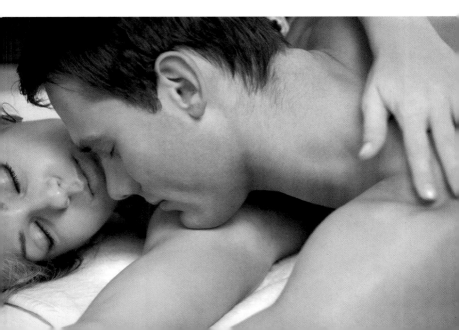

# BEGINNERS' LUST

You'll always remember your first time. But remember, practice makes perfect!

**227** At what age did you start really being interested in the opposite sex?

**228** How did you first learn about sex?

**229** Did you have any crazy misconceptions?

**230** Who did you lose your virginity to?

**231** When and where did you lose your virginity?

**232** If you could go back in time, would you change the circumstances of your first sexual encounter?

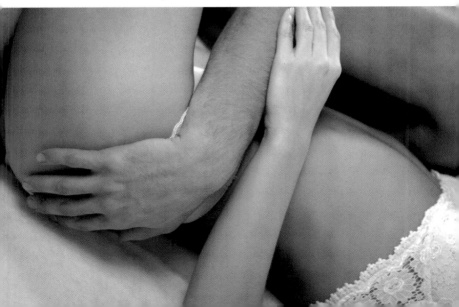

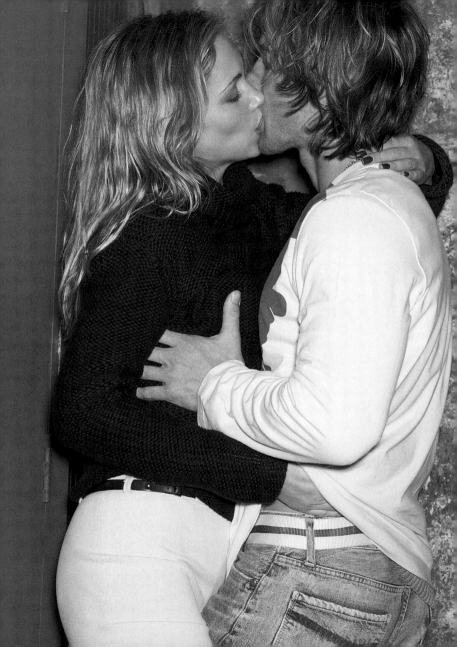

# DO YOU? DO ME!

These quivering questions will help you explore the erotic solutions needed in order to make each other deliriously happy, both in and out of bed.

**233**   Do you want to touch ourselves before we pleasure each other?

**234**   Do you want me to be the aggressor more often?

**235**   Do you ever have any erotic dreams of me? What happens?

**236**   Do you like having your nipples pinched? How hard?

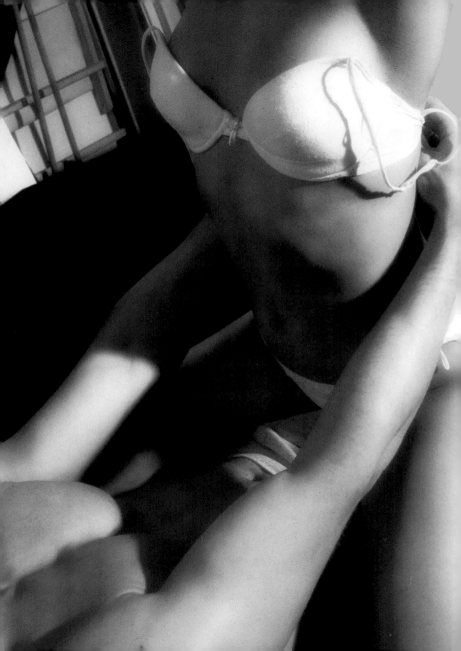

# EROTIC EXTREMES

Discussing our most extreme sex scenarios will not only bring us closer, we'll enjoy setting some new world records of our own.

237   What is the dirtiest escapade you've ever experienced in bed?

238   Which of your fantasies do you think is the naughtiest?

239   What is the greatest wet and wild aquatic adventure you can think of?

240   What is the craziest place you've had sex?

**241** What would be the perfect sexual experience for you?

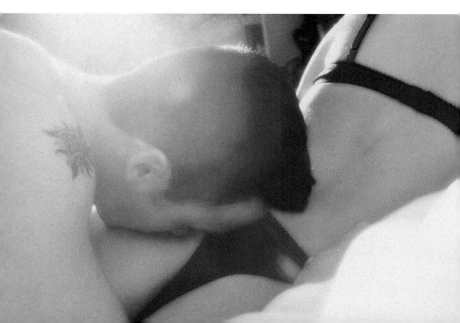

# WANNA EAT OUT?

Let's curb our appetites with a little taste of each other. Knowing exactly what we're hungry for will be a satisfying dessert!

**242** If I wanted to, would you let me put whipped cream anywhere?

**243** What is your favorite food to incorporate into erotic adventures?

**244** If you feed me ice cream and it drips on my naked body, will you lick it off?

**245** What is your aphrodisiac of choice?

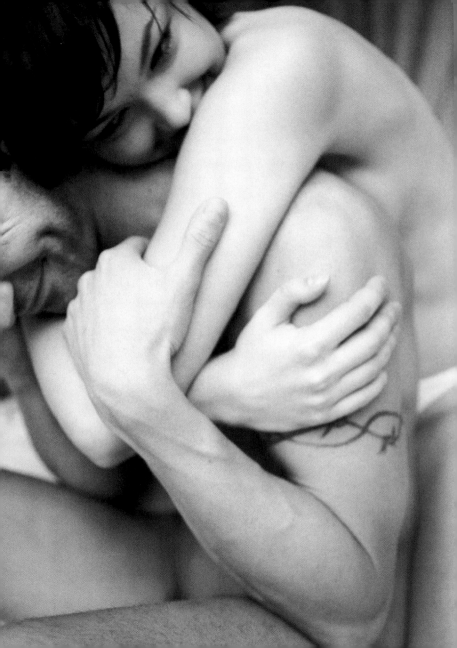

# NAKED EXHIBITIONS

These art-related questions will transform our sex still life into an artistic movement all our own.

**246** Would you consider piercing a part of your body besides your ears?

**247** Which body part would you like me to have pierced?

**248** If you could pick out a tattoo for me, what would it be and where would you put it?

**249** Would you ever tattoo my name on the place I love best?

**250** Which body part would you like me to decorate with a love bite?

**251** Would you like to experiment with body paint? Finger painting or air-brush?

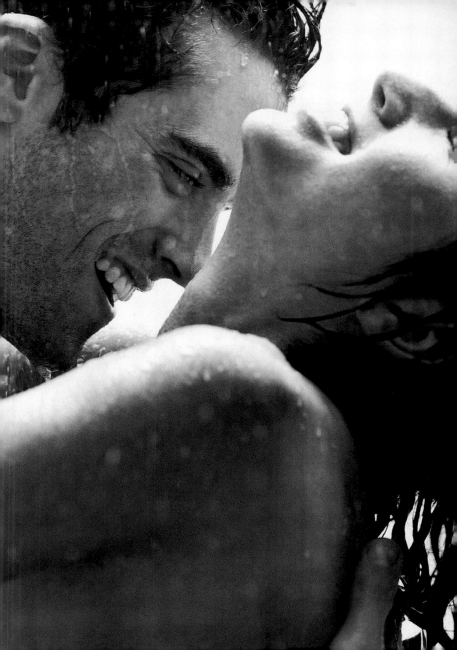

# MATERIAL FUN

Keep the lights on, but take my clothes off—or maybe it'll be hotter if we keep them on!

**252**  What's the most fun you've ever had with your clothes on?

**253**  How about with your clothes off?

**254**  What is your favorite article of clothing that I wear?

**255**  Would you wear my panties/boxers to work?

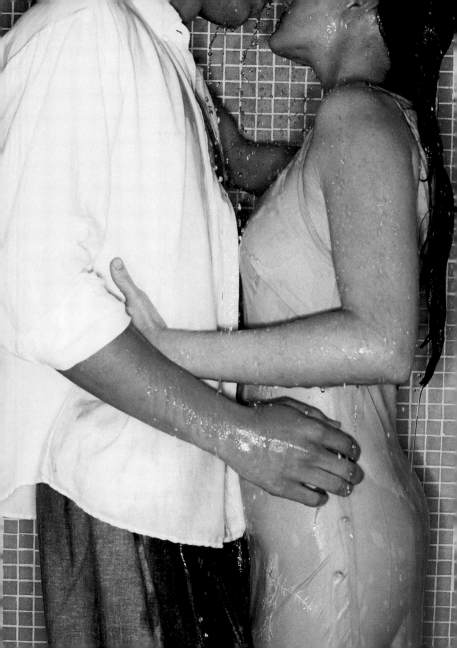

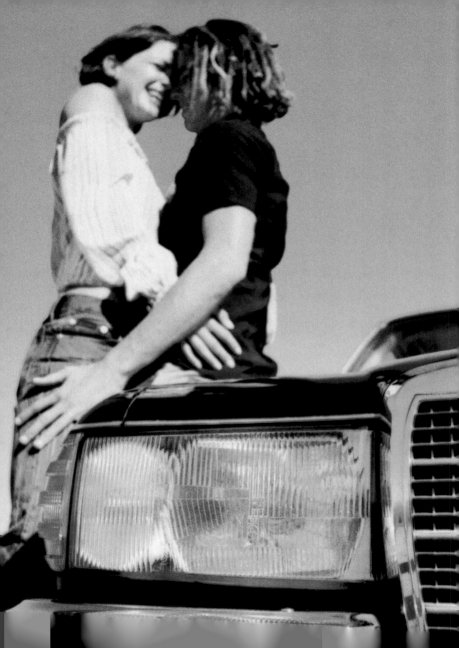

# SEXUAL STATISTICS

Want to be above par? Answer these questions and I'll give you an A-plus in statistics and anatomy.

**256** How would you describe your sexual personality?

**257** How would you describe mine?

**258** What is the best sex advice you've ever gotten?

**259** What is the best sex advice you've ever given?

260    What is the worst sex advice you've ever gotten?

261    Do you consider yourself more or less sensual than other people?

262    Do you think you need sex more or less often than the average person?

263    Do you think we have sex more often than the average couple?

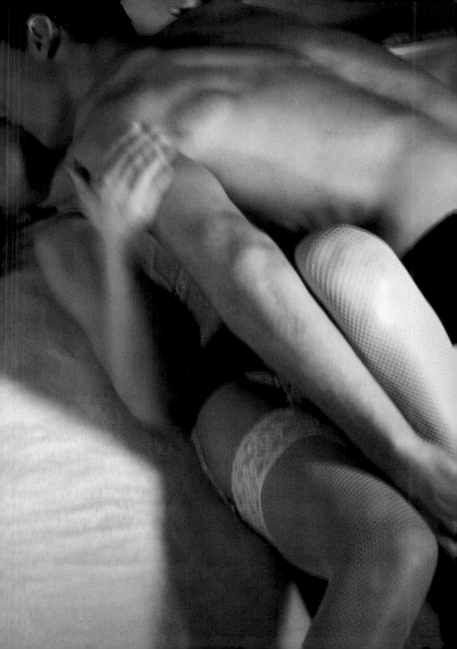

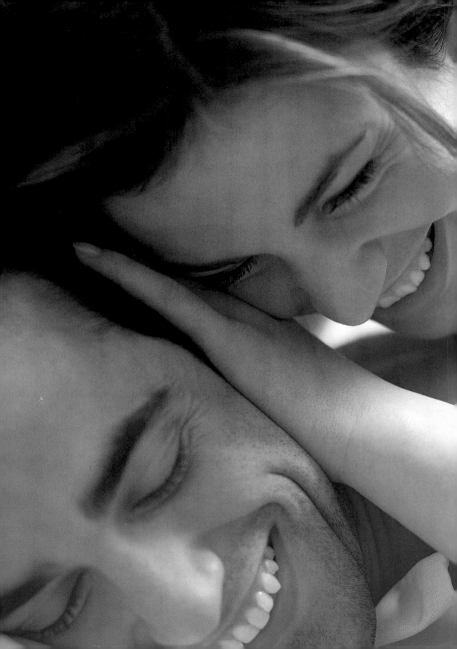

# GIVE ME MOREPLAY

Discussing what we need from each other not only gets us what we want, but hearing the naked truth will make you bare more than just your soul.

**264** What is your favorite foreplay act to receive?

**265** What is your favorite foreplay act to give?

**266** Are there any areas of you that I neglect during sex?

**267** Are there any areas of you that you want me to stay away from?

**268** What is the sexiest thing that I do with my tongue?

**269** Will you massage my back for at least fifteen minutes? You can slip into whatever you want afterward!

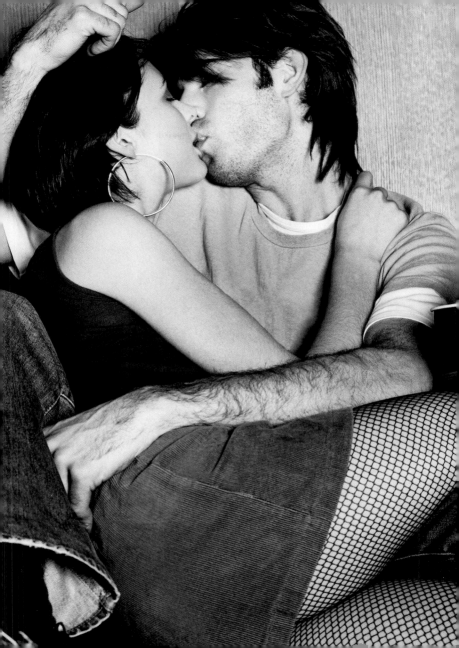